TABLE OF CONTENTS

PROTEIN RECIPES

Shaklee Soy Protein

Imagine a food that can:

- Provide the protein quality of a steak without the fat

- Increase your energy

- Help prevent top cancer killers in men and women (breast, prostate, colon, lung)

- Help prevent top cancer killers in men and women (breast, prostate, colon, lung)

- Reduce the risk of osteoporosis

- Improve hormonal balance

- Support blood sugar management

- And much much more

Pancakes

Combine six tbsp. Instant Protein Soy Mix and one cup pancake mix. Add an additional 3/4 cup milk and follow directions on the box.
Makes 3 servings

MUFFINS

Add 9 1/2 tbsp. Instant Protein Soy Mix to a 19 1/2 oz. box of muffin mix. Increase water by an additional 1/2 cup and follow directions on box.
Makes 12 servings.
Note- When using this product cooking at a lower heat and increasing liquid are recommended.

FOURTEEN KARAT WHEAT PROTEIN BREAKFAST CAKE
For the cake:
16 tbsp. Instant Protein Soy Mix
Two cups sugar
One cup olive oil
Five eggs
One tsp. vanilla
Three cups grated carrots (about three carrots)
Two cups wheat flour
Two tsp. baking soda
Two tsp. cinnamon
1/2 tsp. salt
One cup raisins
One cup chopped walnuts or pecans

For the optional topping:
1/2 cup Shaklee Fibre Plan Daily Crunch
1/2 cup quick cooking oats
1/2 cup brown sugar
1/4 olive oil

METHOD

Preheat oven to 350F. Coat a Bundt pan with non-sticking cooking spray then lightly flour.

In a large bowl beat together sugar and olive oil. Add eggs one at a time, beating after each addition.

Add vanilla, mixing well. Stir in carrots. In a smaller bowl mix together flour, Instant Protein Soy Mix, baking soda, cinnamon and salt. Stir into wet ingredients mixing well. Stir into raisins and nuts.
If making the topping, combine 3/4 of the cake batter with topping ingredients.
Spread topping evenly into the bottom of the Bundt pan then cover with remaining cake batter. If not making the topping, pour batter into the cake pan.
Bake for 60 minutes or until toothpick inserted in middle comes out clean.
Cool 10 minutes, then remove from pan and cool completely.
Makes 14 servings.

180 Protein Pancakes

Combine 1/2 banana smashed well, 2 egg whites that you've given a good scramble, and 2 tbsp. unsweetened almond milk. Stir in 2 scoops vanilla 180 mix and add a little more almond milk as needed. Heat a griddle on medium low, spray with cooking spray and cook as you would regular pancakes. They'll dry out around the edges when they are ready to flip. Serve with fresh berries or apples.

CHIA/HEMP HEART PUDDING/PORRIDGE

In a one pint (2 cup) jar with a lid, add the following:
Four tbsp. hemp hearts
Two tbsp. chia seeds
One tsp. to one tbsp. cinnamon and a handful of raisins.
1/4 cup coconut

Two level tbsp. of Shaklee Soy Protein (vanilla)
Add one cup of water. Put the lid on and shake well
and put in the refrigerator overnight.
In the morning. Breakfast or lunch is ready. Eat
cold.

CHEESE STRATA

This recipe is a great dish for a crowd. You make
it entirely the night before and bake it in the
morning or just before serving.
You can bake it ahead and reheat it if you are
taking it to a friend's house or serving it on a
buffet table for a catering job.
It is healthy and tastes great!
Cuts into six large pieces, approximately five
inches square or into eight smaller pieces.
Four whole organic eggs plus four eggs whites (or
use six whole eggs).
2 1/2 cups 2% milk or regular soy milk, mixed with
three scoops of Soy Protein
Salt and pepper to taste.
8 oz. (2 cups) shredded light cheddar cheese
4 oz. (one cup) light Swiss cheese
Four 1/4 inch small slices of French bread
One tbsp. finely chopped parsley
Organic basil pesto.

METHOD

Mix the whole eggs and egg whites together and add
the milk/protein powder mixture but reserve a half
cup, salt and pepper and parsley. Butter a large
baking pan. Arrange half of the cheese and bread
slices in the pan and pour the egg-milk mixture on
top. To the half cup reserved milk mixture, add
about three tbsp. freshly made pesto and pour on
top. Sprinkle with the remaining cheese and cover.
You may save the remaining cheese to sprinkle on
just before baking. Refrigerate overnight and bake

the next day.
Bake in a glass 13 x9 inch pan at 325F in a water bath for 45-55 minutes depending on doneness. Test to see if the center is cooked. May be reheated.
Note: You may add a pre-cooked sausage meat or ham. Cook the ham slice also and cut into cubes. I use soy milk but it tastes great with regular milk too. If using whole eggs, use 6-8 as it depends on how solid you want this.

CONNIE'S FRENCH TOAST
Four slices whole wheat bread
One large egg
Three egg whites
Two tbsp. Shaklee's Instant Protein Soy Powder
One tbsp. unsalted butter, melted
Your choice of maple syrup or honey
Separate the three eggs and use only the whites. In an 8 inch square glass baking pan, add the egg whites, the whole egg, and beat in the protein powder until mixed and add the butter.
Heat an electric non-stick skillet or griddle to 350F. Dip the bread slices in the egg mixture and cook until the pieces are slightly brown, and turn it over to cook the other side.
Serve with a small amount of maple syrup, Canadian bacon rounds, fresh fruit and tea, and don't forget the water.

CORN MUFFINS
These muffins come from a 6 muffin mix. They are easy but you control what you put in the batter to make a healthier muffin.
One packet corn muffin mix.
One large egg
Four tbsp. Shaklee's Instant Protein Soy Mix.
1/3 cup milk, plus two tbsp. either 2% milk, or light Soy milk
One tbsp. corn oil

Preheat the oven to 400F.
Butter six medium muffin tins. You can use paper liners sprayed with Canola oil.
Mix the protein powder with the muffin mix. In a separate bowl, beat the egg with the milk and oil, and gently stir it into the muffin mixture.

Scoop out the mixture with an ice cream scoop. Bake for 15-16 minutes or until just lightly browned. When the top springs back, the muffins are done. Remove to a dish and serve slightly warm with honey.
Note: You may make any muffin like this, and Blueberry muffins are especially good made this way.

WAFFLES
Two cups whole wheat flour
One cup oatmeal (or 1/2 cup oatmeal and 1/2 cup oat bran)
1/2 cup to one cup flax meal
One block soft tofu (optional)
One egg (optional)
Two tbsp. brown sugar
One tsp. salt
One tsp. soda
Four to six scoops (tbsp.) Shaklee soy mix
Five to six cups water or milk- add water to make a thin batter

Mix thoroughly with electric mixer before cooking in a waffle pan. This mixture thickens quickly because of the oatmeal and flax meal but works ok if made into waffles--more water can be added as needed.
The mixture would not work as well for pancakes. These hearty waffles will keep you feeling "FULL" for hours.

BLUEBERRY PROTEIN PANCAKES

Makes 8 pancakes
One cup flour
One tbsp. sugar
Two tsp. baking powder
1/8 tsp. salt
One tbsp. dried egg white
One or two scoops Shaklee Instant Protein Soy Mix
3/4 cup milk, plus 2-4 tbsp. milk
*hint you need to add more milk because of the soy.
One egg lightly beaten
One tbsp. Canola Oil or melted unsalted butter
2/3 fresh blueberries.

METHOD

Mix the dry ingredients and the wet ingredients separately. Pour the wet into the dry ingredients. Do not stir too much. A few lumps are fine.
You will need a bit more milk, depending on how much protein you use.
Add blueberries. Cook at 350F in a square electric skillet and turn over when bubbles appear. You may use a bit more oil to give the crunch to the pancakes and to get a bit more browning.
These are thick, light and deliciously healthy for you and your family, and good anytime. Complete meal in itself or with soy sausages or crisp bacon and fruit.

JOEY'S SOY PROTEIN BREAKFAST PATTIES
Six tbsp. Instant Protein Soy Mix
Two 6 oz. cans tuna in water, drained
Five tbsp. mayonnaise
One egg or egg white
1/4 cup breadcrumbs
Salt and pepper to taste

METHOD

In a medium bowl mix all ingredients together
Form into patties about 3 inches in diameter
Lightly coat a large skillet with olive oil
On medium heat cook patties about 4 inches per
Side until lightly browned.

BLUEBERRY BLISS

Two scoops Shaklee Vanilla 180
Eight oz. non-fat/light soy milk
1/4 cup blueberries
1/4 banana
Ice

MOCHA LATTE

One scoop Shaklee Coffee Latte 180
One scoop Chocolate Shaklee 180
Eight oz. / non-fat/light-soy milk
Two-four drops coffee extract
Ice

PINA COLADA

Two scoops Shaklee vanilla 180
Eight oz. non-fat/light soy milk
1/2 cup pineapple chunks
1/2 tsp. vanilla extract
Ice

BERRY BLAST

One scoop Shaklee vanilla 180
One scoop Shaklee strawberry 180
Eight oz. non-fat/light soy milk

1/2 cup frozen mixed berries

SPICED
Two scoops Shaklee vanilla 180
Eight oz. non-fat/light soy milk
1/2 tsp. pumpkin pie spice or cinnamon
Ice

PEANUT BUTTER CUP
Two scoops Shaklee chocolate 180
Eight oz. non-fat light soy milk
One tsp. peanut butter
Ice

JUST PEACHY
Two scoops Shaklee vanilla 180
Eight oz. non-fat/light soy milk
1/2 cup peach slices
Ice

SPICED LATTE
Two scoops Shaklee cafe' latte 180
Eight oz. non-fat/light soy milk
1/2 tsp. pumpkin pie spice
Ice

PUMPKIN PIE
Two scoops Shaklee vanilla 180
Eight oz. non-fat/light soy milk
1/4 tsp. pumpkin pie spice
One cup fresh cooked pumpkin
Ice

ST.PATTY'S PLEASURE
Two scoops Shaklee vanilla 180
One handful of spinach or chard
1/2 cup fresh strawberries
1/2 banana
12 oz. cold water
Ice

HAWAIIAN
Two scoops Shaklee vanilla 180
Eight oz. non-fat/light soy milk
1/2 banana
1/2 cup pineapple chunks
1/2 tsp. coconut extract

CHOCOLATE COVERED BANANA
Two scoops chocolate 180
Eight oz. non-fat/light soy milk
1/2 banana
Ice

STRAWBERRY CHARD
Two scoops Shaklee strawberry 180
A handful of red chard
4 oz. canned pumpkin
One inch fresh ginger
Three frozen strawberries
12 oz. water
Ice

FRENCH CHRISTIANA
Two scoops Shaklee vanilla 180
Eight oz. non-fat/light soy milk
1/2 tsp. ground ginger
1/8 tsp. cayenne pepper
1/8 tsp. cinnamon
Ice

MINT CHOCOLATE CHIP
Two scoops Shaklee chocolate 180
Eight oz. non-fat/light soy milk
2-4 drops mint extract
Ice

ORANGE CREAM DELIGHT
Two scoops Shaklee vanilla 180
Eight oz. non-fat/light soy milk
4 oz. orange juice

Ice

STRAWBERRY LEMONADE
Two scoops Shaklee strawberry 180
Eight oz. non-fat/light soy milk
Two oz. lemonade
Ice

STRAWBERRY BANANA
Eight oz. non-fat/light soy milk
Three frozen strawberries
1/2 banana
Ice

APPLE PIE IN A GLASS
Six tbsp. Shaklee Chocolate 180
1/2 cup water
1/2 cup unsweetened applesauce
1/2 tsp. cinnamon
1/4 tsp. nutmeg
Four ice cubes
Mix in blender until smooth

APPLE PIE SMOOTHIE
Put in a blender:
Two tbsp. Shaklee Soy Mix or three tbsp. Energizing
Vanilla Soy
One cup either:
Organic unsweetened Vanilla Almond Breeze or
unsweetened Vanilla Coconut milk or unsweetened Soy
milk
One apple
1/2 banana and/or two tbsp. flax seeds
Add filtered water to desired consistency.
Add cinnamon to taste

APRICOT/PEACH PLEASER

One small can of lemonade
One can water
One banana
Four tbsp. Shaklee Vanilla Instant Protein
Six ice cubes
Whirl in blender

BANANA SMOOTHIE
Two-three tbsp. Shaklee Energizing Protein
One cup rice, almond or soy milk
1/4 cup yogurt
Combine in blender

BAVARIAN MINT HOT COCOA
One cup rice, almond or soy milk
One serving Shaklee Chocolate 180
Peppermint extract
Warm milk, add 180...add extract to taste

BERRY COOLER
Eight oz. plain yogurt
1/2 carton frozen strawberries or 8-10 fresh berries
Two tbsp. Shaklee Soy Protein
1/4-1/2 cup water
Mix all except water in blender.
Add cold water to desired consistency or freeze and eat
with a spoon.

BIG APPLE
One apple
One medium apple, chopped
Three tbsp. Shaklee Vanilla Soy Protein
Dash of nutmeg
1/4 tsp. cinnamon
Four-eight ice cubes
Combine in blender
Extremely refreshing on a hot day!

CAFE-SOY MOCHA

To one cup of soy or rice milk add:
Two tbsp. Shaklee Soy Protein (cocoa) or chocolate 180
One tbsp. Caf-lib
Whip in the blender
Delicious!

CHOCOLATE DATE SHAKE
16 oz. milk
Four tbsp. Shaklee Cocoa Soy Protein
Six dates cut up
Two-three ice cubes
1/2 fresh or frozen bananas (optional)
Place all ingredients in blender.
Whirl at least one minute
Enjoy!

CHOCOLATE LOVERS DELIGHT
One cup chocolate milk (rice, soy or dairy)
Three tbsp. Shaklee Cocoa Soy Protein
1/4 tsp. vanilla
Dash of cinnamon
3-4 ice cubes
Combine in blender

CHOCOLATE MONKEY
One banana
1 1/2 cups milk (soy or rice)
Two tbsp. Shaklee Soy Protein (cocoa)
1 1/2 tbsp. honey
Combine all ingredients in blender.
Blend until smooth.

COCOA BANANA FLIP
Six tbsp. Shaklee Protein (cocoa)
3/4 cup water
1/2 cup fresh or frozen banana
Four ice cubes
Dash of cinnamon
Mix in blender until smooth

COCOA BANANA SMOOTHIE
1/2 banana
Three tbsp. Cocoa Soy Protein
1/2 cup milk (rice/soy/reg)
1/2 cup water
One tsp. Vanilla extract
Two-three ice cubes

COCOA VANILLA TREAT
3/4 cup water
1/2 cup milk (rice/soy/reg)
Three tbsp. Vanilla or Chocolate Soy Protein
One tsp. Vanilla extract
Two-three ice cubes
Optional- dash of cinnamon

COOL GOLD
Two cups apple juice
Two tbsp. frozen orange juice concentrate
Five ice cubes
Four tbsp. Shaklee Vanilla Instant Soy Protein
Place in blender for a few minutes
Enjoy!

CRANBERRY FIESTA
One cup cranberry juice
Three tbsp. Vanilla Soy Protein
1/2 pineapple
Two-three ice cubes

FROSTY ISLAND SHAKE
One cup buttermilk
One cup crushed pineapple (in unsweetened juice)
Six tbsp. Vanilla Soy Protein
One tbsp. lemon juice
Eight ice cubes
Combine in blender

FROSTY PEACH MELBA

Six tbsp. Vanilla Soy Protein
3/4 cup water
1/2 cup diced fresh peaches
1/4 frozen red raspberries
Four ice cubes
Mix in blender

FRUIT PUNCH
Two cups apple juice
Three tbsp. frozen orange juice concentrate
Two tbsp. Shaklee Vanilla Soy Protein
One banana
Seven ice cubes
Combine all ingredients in blender.
Blend until smooth
Enjoy

FRUIT SLUSH
1/2 cup frozen strawberries
1/2 banana
Two tbsp. Shaklee Soy Protein
One ice cube
One tbsp. crushed pineapple or 1/2 fresh apple
Mix in blender until smooth

GREEN SMOOTHIE
Two cups water in Vita Mix
One small banana or one cup berries
One scoop Shaklee 180
One scoop Physique
Two handfuls black kale

GREEN SMOOTHIE
1 1/2 cup strawberries
3/4 cup pineapple
1/2 banana or fruit of your choice
One avocado
1 1/2 cups water, add more if you want it thicker
Six-eight tbsp. Shaklee Protein Powder

One large handful baby spinach
Two large handfuls organic greens
Makes three 8 oz. serving

INSTANT PROTEIN DRINK
One cup of your favorite juice
1/2 cup water
One serving Instant Protein
Optional-one tsp. vanilla, almond or lemon extract

JIM BURKE'S POWER DRINK
Two cans instant protein
One can of physique
1/2 can Fiber Plan
Mix together-shake 1/4 or more in water

HOT CHOCOLATE HEALTHY

Two cups milk or water
Two scoops Shaklee Chocolate 180 Smoothie Mix
Two scoops Shaklee Cocoa Protein
Heat milk or water to near boiling point and pour into
blender. Add proteins.
Whirl two seconds and pour into mugs.
Optional; Add small scoop whipped cream.

"Julius" Smoothie
 One cup orange juice
 Two scoops protein
Three or four ice cubes.
Blend in the magic bullet or blender.
This is very refreshing and gets you going.

Mango Shake
Two heaping tsp. of Shaklee Vanilla Protein

One half cup chopped fresh mango or fruit of your choice
One cup filtered water
Four or five ice cubes
Blend until fresh and enjoy a taste of the tropics

Mango Orange Smoothie
Blend one mango peeled and one orange peeled.
One half cup Shaklee Vanilla Protein
Add a cup of ice
Blend and enjoy!

Mystery Drink
¾ cups water
½ cup juice (apple, cranberry, raspberry or cherry).
3 tbsp. Shaklee Cocoa Soy Protein
2-3 ice cubes
Optional- 2-3 tbsp. vanilla yogurt

Numero Uno

In a blender place the following:
16 oz. water
½ cup orange juice concentrate
2 tbsp. Shaklee Fiber Plan
4 tbsp. Shaklee Vanilla Instant Protein
5 frozen strawberries
Blend well and enjoy!

Orange Julie
Blend until smooth and frothy:
4 TBSP. Shaklee Vanilla Meal Shake
2 tbsp. Shaklee Vanilla Protein
3 ½ cups orange juice
3 ice cubes

Orange Julius
½ cup orange juice

½ cup milk (soy, rice or regular milk)
3 tbsp. Shaklee Vanilla Soy Protein
2-3 ice cubes
Combine in blender

Orange Splash

1 cup orange juice
½ banana
3 tbsp. Shaklee Vanilla Soy Protein
2-3 ice cubes
Combine in blender

Orange Banana Breeze
Combine in Blender:
2 ½ cups milk (soy, rice, or dairy
3 tbsp. Shaklee Vanilla Soy Protein
One banana
2 tbsp. honey (optional)
1/3 cup orange juice

Peanut Butter Cupcake
In Blender mix the following;
Two cups milk of your choice
Four tbsp. Shaklee 180 Meal Shake
Two tbsp. Shaklee Instant Soy Protein
Three ice cubes
Three tbsp. creamy peanut butter
Enjoy!

Peanut Butter Fudge Shake
Three tbsp. Chocolate 180 Smoothie
One cup soy or rice milk
1 ½ tbsp. creamy peanut butter
Combine all ingredients in butter until smooth
A delicious nourishing drink.

Pina Colada
½ cup pineapple juice
¼ cup crushed ice

One ripe banana
Two scoops Vanilla Soy Protein- Energizing or 180
Smoothie
 Lower Calorie Version
½ cup pineapple juice
½ cup water
½ cup crushed ice
½ banana
Two scoops protein powder

Pineapple Delight
1/3 cup pineapple juice
¾ cup cold water
Three tbsp. Vanilla Soy Protein
One tsp. fresh orange juice
2-3 ice cubes
Optional- add fresh pineapple

Pineapple Pleasure
½ cup Soy Milk
½ cup fresh clean water
Two scoops Shaklee 180 Vanilla Shake Mix
Pineapple chunks cut from a quarter pineapple slice
Slice of fresh thinly cut ginger-optional
5-6 ice cubes
Blend the soy milk and vanilla protein powder first
then add the pineapple and the ginger with the ice
cubes.
If you omit the ginger you could use nutmeg instead.

PUMPKIN PIE IN A GLASS
Six tbsp. Shaklee Vanilla 180 Mix
One tsp, pumpkin pie spice
One cup milk (almond or rice).
Four ice cubes
Mix in blender

Raspberry Ice
¼ cup fresh or frozen raspberries
Three tbsp. Shaklee Vanilla Protein

One cup rice (almond, soy, or rice).
½ cup vanilla ice cream
One tbsp. honey
½ tsp. vanilla
Blend until smooth

Slim Jim Drink
One serving Shaklee Vanilla 180 Mix
One cup or more water
Optional- dash cinnamon or nutmeg

Tutti Fruiti
½ cup orange juice
¾ cup water
Several berries
½ cup peach or nectarines
2-3 strawberries
Three tbsp. Shaklee Vanilla Soy Protein
2-3 ice cubes
Optional- vanilla or almond extract

Tropical Treat
One cup of Doles Juice (pineapple, banana or orange)
½ cup water
Four strawberries
½ banana
2-3 tbsp. Shaklee Vanilla Soy Protein
2-3 Ice cubes

Very Berry Drink
Four strawberries
Several blueberries and or raspberries
½ banana
¾ water
½ cup apple juice
Three tbsp. Shaklee Vanilla Soy Protein
2-3 ice cubes
Blend well

Yogurt Julius

¼ plain yogurt
¾ cup orange juice
½ cup water
Two tbsp. vanilla extract
Three tbsp. Vanilla Soy Protein
2-3 ice cubes

Almond Butter Nut Chews
½ cup of each butter and almond butter
½ cup chopped pecans
½ cup chopped Brazil nuts
½ cup coconut
1/3 cup raisins
Three cups course rolled oats
One cup Shaklee Soy Protein Powder
Mix first three ingredients until smooth.
Combine all other ingredients
Press mixture into a 9x9 inch pan.
Refrigerate and cut into squares or bars.

Carob Logs
Mix the following ingredients
½-3/4 cup liquid honey
½ cup skim milk powder
1 ½ cup organic smooth peanut butter
One tsp. vanilla
½ cup unsweetened carob powder
One cup Shaklee Cocoa Protein powder
Two cup mixed nuts (walnuts, pecans, sunflower seeds.
½ cup unsalted butter
Add more water or butter if too dry or more protein if too wet.
Roll into four logs. Wrap and freeze. To serve, remove from freezer and slice.

Chocolate Almond Butter Slices
½ cup butter
½ cup raw honey
1/3 cup Shaklee Physique Whey Powder

One tsp. vanilla
½ cup cocoa
One cup Shaklee Soy Protein
One cup each chopped pecans and almonds.

Mix butter, honey, Physique, and vanilla until smooth.
Next combine cocoa and soy protein and blend.
Add nuts and first mixture.
Add more protein if too wet.
Divide batter into two parts. Roll in wax paper into logs. Wrap and freeze.
To serve, remove from freezer, slice immediately and serve.

Crunchy Delights
Equal amounts of honey, protein supplement, (can add cocoa powder)
Natural crunchy peanut butter
Post grape nuts
Mix together. Form into small balls and roll in crushed nuts.

Fiber Nuggets
2/3 cup Shaklee Protein Soy Mix or Vanilla or Instant Soy
One cup old fashioned oats, uncooked
One cup AL bran buds
¾ cup honey
One cup peanut butter
2 ½ tsp. vanilla
2/3 cups raisins or carob chips
Combine oats, protein and all bran buds in large bowl and set aside
Bring honey to a boil on stovetop.
Remove from heat and stir in peanut butter and vanilla until smooth. Immediately add honey mixture and mix well. Stir in raisins and press into 8 x 8 inch pan square pan. If you choose carob chips instead of raisins refrigerate for 20-25 minutes first, then stir in carob chips and press into 8 x8 inch pan.

Refrigerate until firm. Cut into small squares and serve. Store bars refrigerator in airtight container.

Fiber Protein Bars
Mix the following and heat until soft.
One cup peanut butter-preferably crunchy
¾ cup honey
Stir in 2/3 cup Shaklee Protein
Add two cups organic cereal
Press into 9 x13 inch glass dish
Top with 12 oz. bag chocolate chips and put under broiler, until it just gets warm and then spread around evenly.

Healthy Chewy Bars
¼ cup butter
½ cup molasses
½ cup peanut butter
These are approximate amounts. If you wish to make more than just increase the liquid. Also experiment with using either honey or brown rice syrup and with or without peanut butter. Melt ingredients in a large sauce pan.

Then the fun begins. Add whatever you desire. Add until mixture is thick and blobby.
Sesame seeds, sunflower seeds, peanuts, pumpkin seeds, chopped almonds, unsweetened coconut. Shaklee protein powder, any flavor.
All ingredients should be raw and unsalted.
Put mixture into a glass pan (can butter it a bit to make the squares easier to remove). Cut into squares and refrigerate. When cooled (approx.) one hour remove from pan. Ready to eat. Keep leftover in the fridge or freezer. Enjoy!

No Bake Healthy Cookies
One cup honey
¼ cup butter
¼ cup milk

¼ cup cocoa
Mix these ingredients in a pot and bring to a boil over low heat.
Add one tsp, vanilla
One cup Shaklee vanilla or cocoa protein powder.
¾ cup shredded coconut
¾ cup organic cereal
One cup quick cooking oats
Mix altogether and drop by spoon onto a cookie sheet lined with wax paper.

Peanut Butter Chocolate Chip Bars
One cup Shaklee Instant Protein Soy Mix
One cup old fashioned oats- uncooked
1 ½ cups Shaklee Fiber Plan Daily Crunch
¾ cup honey
One cup peanut butter
2 ½ tsp. vanilla or 1 tsp. almond extract
½ cup chocolate chips

Combine oats, protein and fiber in large bowl. Set aside. Bring honey to a light boil on stovetop. Remove from heat and stir in peanut butter and vanilla until smooth. Immediately add honey mixture to dry mixture until well incorporated. Refrigerate for 10 minutes. Stir in chocolate chips and press into an 8 x 8 inch square pan. Refrigerate 20 minutes or until firm.
Cut into 12 bars. Chill and serve.
Store bars in airtight container.
You could also use 1/3 cup raisins and 1/3 cup roasted almonds or pecans.
When using chocolate chips, melt a handful of chocolate chips and a scoop of peanut butter and spread over the top.

Peanut Butter Slices
One cup natural peanut butter
2 ½ tbsp. non-fat dry milk

Three tbsp. Shaklee Protein Supplement
½ cup raisins, dried cranberries or chocolate chips
Two tbsp. honey
Blend all ingredients and shape into a log.
Chill and serve.

Protein Balls
 Mix in bowl:
Two cups quick oatmeal (or grind old fashioned oats).
½ cup of one of the following: raisins or chopped dates
or carob chips
½ cup of one of the following: chopped walnuts or
sunflower seeds or almonds
½ cup Shaklee Cocoa Energizing Soy Protein or the
Vanilla Soy Protein Mix
½ cup unsweetened coconut to roll the balls in
Cream together:
½ cup maple syrup or a bit less honey
½ cup fresh ground without sugar peanut butter
1/3 cup warm water
Mix two groups together and roll into small balls. Roll
in unsweetened coconut if you wish.

Protein Balls
One cup Shaklee Soy Mix
½ cup oats- quick or slow cooking
One or two cups granola of your choice
½ cup pumpkin seeds
¾ cup honey
One cup peanut butter
Two to three tsp. vanilla
2/3 cup chocolate chips or raisins
After mixing ingredients, roll into balls and then roll
balls into fine coconut, sweetened or unsweetened
These can be refrigerated or frozen for a few weeks if
desired.

Protein Bars
½ cup organic sunflower butter
1/3 cup coconut oil
½ cup honey
Melt on low heat:

Then add:
One tsp. vanilla
Two cups crunched cereal
One cup protein powder
Press into a 9 x 12 inch pan.
Top with one cup chocolate chips
Put under broiler until the melt, then spread evenly
over the bars.

Snicker Snackers
1/3 cup each sunflower seeds, pumpkin seeds, and sesame
seeds
½ cup honey or less
½ cup nut butter (peanut, almond or soy)
½ cup Shaklee Chocolate or Vanilla Soy Protein
¼ cup ground flaxseed (these grind best in a coffee
grinder)
¼ cup unsweetened coconut (optional)
Grind the seeds first in a food processor. Combine
ingredients in a bowl.
Pat into an 8 x 8 inch square pan or form into small
balls (if mixture is too soft refrigerate or half an
hour).
Optional- roll each ball into coconut or carob to coat,
Keep refrigerated.

PEANUT BUTTER BALLS

One cup peanut butter chunky, almond or tahini.
One cup Shaklee's Energizing Vanilla Protein.
1/2 cup honey
One cup granola or any kind of ground nuts.
Unsweetened coconut, currants, raisins, crushed Honey
Nut Cereal
Mix to a thick but not sticky consistency.

Add more honey and more Protein as desired.
Roll in small balls. A small cookie dough baller works
well with this.
Coat with sesame seed, ground or chopped nuts, coconut,
cocoa or have them plain.
Freezes well.

ALMOND BUTTER NUT CHEWS

1/2 cup butter
1/2 cup almond butter
1 tsp. vanilla
1/2 cup chopped pecans
1/2 cup chopped Brazil nuts
1/2 cup raisins
1/2 cup coconut
Three cups coarse rolled oats
One cup Soy Protein Powder
Mix first three ingredients until smooth.
Combine all other ingredients.
Press mixture into a 9x9 inch pan
Refrigerate. Cut into bars or squares.

CAROB LOGS
Mix the following ingredients
1/2-3/4 cups liquid honey
1/2 cup skim milk powder-preferably non instant
1 1/2 cups organic smooth peanut butter
1 tsp. vanilla
1/2 tsp. unsweetened Carob Powder
One cup Shaklee Cocoa Protein Powder or Shaklee
Chocolate Protein Powder
Two cups mixed nuts and seeds (walnuts, pecans,
sunflower seeds, etc.
1/2 cup unsalted butter
Add more water or butter if too dry or more protein if
too wet. Roll into four logs. Wrap and freeze.
To serve, remove from freezer and slice.

CHOCOLATE ALMOND BUTTER SLICES

1/2 cup each butter and honey.
1/2 cup Physique Whey Protein Powder
One tsp. vanilla
1/2 cup cocoa

One cup Shaklee Soy Protein
One cup chopped nuts
One cup almonds
Mix butter, honey, Physique, and vanilla until smooth.
Next combine protein and cocoa and blend
Add nuts and first mixture
Add more protein powder if too wet
Divide batter into four parts
Roll into logs in wax paper and freeze.
To serve, unwrap from freezer and slice.

CRUNCHY DELIGHTS

Equal amounts of honey, protein supplement (can add
cocoa powder)
Natural Crunchy Peanut Butter
Post Grape Nuts
Mix together. Roll into small balls and roll in crushed
nuts.

MIXED BERRY BAR

Ten tablespoons Instant Protein Soy Mix
One cup Shaklee Fiber Plan Daily Crunch
One cup Post® Grape Nut® Flakes*
One cup rolled oats
1 1/2 cups dried fruit mix (cranberries, raisins, or
any other dried fruit)
1 1/2 teaspoon cinnamon

1/3 cup sliced almonds
One cup honey
1/3 cup orange juice concentrate
Combine Instant Protein Soy Mix, Shaklee Fiber Plan
Daily Mix, cereal, oats, dried fruit mix, cinnamon, and

almonds; set aside. Bring honey and orange juice concentrate to a boil on stovetop and remove from heat.

MOLASSES HONEY GINGER COOKIES

1/2 cup shortening
1/2 cup sugar
1/4 cup molasses
1/4 cup honey
1 egg yolk
1 1/2 cups flour
One teaspoon baking powder
1/2 teaspoon baking soda
1/2 teaspoon salt
1/2 tablespoon cinnamon
1 teaspoon ground cloves
1 teaspoon ground ginger
1/2 teaspoon ground nutmeg
  Preheat oven to 350°F.
Cream together shortening, sugar, molasses, and honey. Add the egg yolk and mix well. In a separate bowl, sift together the remaining ingredients. Stir flour mixture into shortening mixture. Form dough into a disc shape, cover with plastic wrap, and refrigerate for at least 1 hour.
On a lightly floured surface, roll dough out ¼ inch thick. Use more flour if dough is sticky.
  Use cookie cutters to make shapes and transfer onto lightly greased cookie sheets. Bake 8-10 minutes or until edges are set and middles are still soft. Do not over bake.
Let the cookies cool on the baking sheets until they are firm, then transfer to a rack to cool completely. Decorate with confectioners' icing sugar and Shaklee Fiber Plan Daily Crunch if desired.
Makes about 2 dozen medium-size cookies

COOKIES

Add 13 tablespoons Instant Protein Soy Mix to a package of dry cookie mix (1 lb 1.5 oz. to 1 lb 4 oz.-package). Add an additional 1/3 cup milk and follow instructions on package. Makes 18 servings

One tbsp. Canola Oil or melted unsalted butter
2/3 fresh blueberries

METHOD
Mix the dry ingredients and the wet ingredients separately. Pour the wet into the dry ingredients. Do not stir too much. A few lumps are fine.
You will need a bit more milk, depending on how much protein you use.
Add blueberries. Cook at 350F in a square electric skillet and turn over when bubbles appear. You may use

CHOCOLATE POPSICLES

One cup of milk, soy or almond
Two scoops of Chocolate Soy Protein
Mix well and put into popsicle mould.
Freeze and serve chocolate soy shake with almond or soy milk and then pour that into popsicle mould and give it to the kids for dessert.

CHOCOLATE SILK PIE
CRUST
You may buy all natural product chocolate or vanilla crust or make your own.

FILLING

16 OZ. Silken soft tofu.
One tbsp. honey
Two scoops Shaklee Instant Protein Soy Mix (about four tbsp.).
1 1/2-3 tbsp. powdered egg white
One tsp. vanilla extract
Two cups semi-sweet chocolate chips melted in double boiler
Blend the tofu in a food processor fitted with a steal blade.
Add the remaining ingredients and blend well. Add the chocolate and blend until completely mixed, stopping to scrape down the sides. Pour into the pie crust and refrigerate for at least two hours. Serve each piece with a dab of whipped cream, a mint sprig or raspberries or strawberries.

FRESH BANANA CHEESECAKE
CRUST
1 1/2 cups graham cracker crumbs
Two tbsp. fructose
Six tbsp. melted butter
Mix and press into pie place or mould pan
Chill 45 minutes and fill

FILLING
Sprinkle one package plus one tsp. Knox Gelatin into 1/3 cup of boiling water.
Stir until dissolved.
Add the following items to your blender:
Two tbsp. Shaklee Vanilla Soy Protein
1/4 tsp. vanilla
One package cream cheese
1 1/4 cups mashed banana (about 6 medium)
1/3 cup liquid honey
Whip until well blended. Add your dissolved gelatin and blend again until well blended.
SERVE

HEALTHY NO BAKE FUDGE

Mix in bowl:

One cup peanut, pecan or almond butter
1/2 cup honey or brown rice syrup for less sweetness.
One cup Shaklee Energizing Soy Protein-cocoa flavour
Optional-1/2 cup Shaklee Fibre Plan Daily Crunch
Morsels
Thoroughly combine ingredients
Chill briefly to firm up ingredients
Spoon out and roll into fudge balls or roll fudge in
waxed paper into a log and cut into bite size pieces.
Keep refrigerated for optimum freshness.

PUMPKIN CHEESECAKE

1 1/2 cups graham wafer crumbs
Two tbsp. fructose
Six tbsp. melted butter
Mix and press into pie plate or mould pan. Chill crust
for 45 minutes and then fill.

FILLING

Sprinkle one package plus one tsp. Knox Gelatin into
1/3 cup boiling water.
Stir until dissolved. Add the following ingredients to
your blender:

1/2 cup each yogurt and water
Two tbsp. Shaklee Instant Soy Protein
1/4 tsp. vanilla
One package cream cheese
One 19 oz. canned pumpkin
1/3 cup liquid honey
Two tsp. pumpkin pie spice
Whip until well blended. Add your dissolved gelatin and
whip again until well blended.

SOY PASTRY CRUST
This makes a 9 inch crust using olive oil and may be
made blind which means to make it with weights in it
before using for a pie. It may shrink a bit.

METHOD
3/4 cups flour, unbleached, organic or oat flour
1/4 cup ground textured soy protein, or soy flour, use
Shaklee's Instant Protein Soy Powder
1/4 cup canola oil, plus two-three tbsp. warm water
Pinch of salt
With a mixture combine the flour and protein powder
together. Mix together the water, oil, and salt and add
it slowly to the flour mixture while beating. Beat for
two-three minutes or until it is wet enough for the
dough to stick together.
Roll the dough between two sheets of plastic wrap.
Uncover the top side and place the crust in a 9 inch
pie plate. You could make this in a square pan and
serve it by cutting it into squares. Use this crust for
Zone Pumpkin Pie which follows.

ZONE PUMPKIN PIE
One can 18 oz. pumpkin
One tbsp. cornstarch
1/2 tsp. cinnamon
1/2 tsp. ginger
1/2 tsp. ground cloves
Two scoops Shaklee Instant Protein Soy Mix

One tbsp. honey
One tbsp. unsalted butter, melted
One cup plain soy milk
1/2 cup sugar
Three egg whites, well beaten
3/4 cup walnut halves

METHOD
Sift together sugar, cornstarch, salt, cinnamon,
ginger, cloves and soy protein. Mix this with one can

pumpkin, honey and butter. Stir in the milk. Beat the
egg whites until very light. Stir in 1/4 of the egg
whites into the pumpkin mixture and gently fold the
whites into the base. Pour into an unbaked pie crust,
preferably a soy crust and decorate with walnut halves.

BAKING
Bake the pie at 400F on the bottom shelf for the first
7 minutes. Reduce the heat to 325F and bake for another
35 minutes or until the center is not liquid. You may
bake the pie in a pie plate or square pan without the
crust. But once you have made this pie with the soy
crust, you will not want to make it without the crust.

CRUSTLESS FRENCH APPLE PIE
Preheat oven to 425F
INGREDIENTS

1/2 cup or less sugar
1/4 cup Instant Protein Soy Mix
1/2 tsp. nutmeg
1/2 tsp. cinnamon
Dash of salt
Six cups thinly slices, pared apples

TOPPING
1/4 cup Instant Protein Soy Mix
1/4 cup quick oats
1/4 cup flour
1/4 cup brown sugar
1/2 stick butter, organic if possible

METHOD
Mix sugar, protein, nutmeg, cinnamon and salt.
Stir in apples.
Arrange in a 9" pie plate.
Mix topping ingredients until crumbly.
Add the topping. Lightly cover so the topping doesn't
burn.

Bake 50 minutes

RICOTTA STUFFED SQUASH

Eight tbsp. Instant Protein Soy Mix
Eight large patty pan squash, ends trimmed, halved
horizontally
Two tbsp. olive oil
One small onion, finely chopped
One clove fresh garlic, minced
One 10 oz. package frozen spinach, thawed and squeezed
to remove moisture.
Two eggs
One 15 oz. package low fat ricotta cheese
1/4 cup grated Parmesan cheese
One tbsp. dried Italian herbs
One tbsp. chopped fresh parsley

METHOD

Scoop seeds from squash halves. Steam squash for five
minutes then set aside.
In a medium bowl combine eggs, ricotta, Instant Protein
Soy Mix, Parmesan, parsley and Italian herbs. Set
aside.
Fill each squash with 3-4 tbsp. of stuffing arranging
filled shells in a baking pan.
Bake uncovered for 30 minutes until squash is soft and
stuffing is heated through.
Makes eight servings.

LASAGNA
Six tbsp. Instant Protein Soy Mix
One cup water
Two cups mozzarella cheese, shredded
1/2 lb. lean ground beef

1/2 medium onion, chopped
Two garlic cloves, minced
One cup mushrooms, sliced
One jar (26 oz.) Healthy Choice pasta sauce

1/2 tsp, oregano, dried
1/2 tsp. basil dried
Eight oz. lasagna noodles

METHOD

In a blender combine the Instant Protein Soy Mix, water and ricotta cheese
Blend until smooth. Stir in 1 1/2 cups ricotta cheese and set aside.
Cook lasagna noodles according to package directions. Set aside. Brown ground beef in skillet, draining fat and reserving meat.
In the same skillet sauté onion, garlic and mushroom until softened. Add pasta sauce, reserved meat, oregano and basil. Stir until well combined.
In a 13 x 9 inch baking pan spread a small amount of pasta sauce in bottom of pan. Place three of the noodles in pan, layer sauce and ricotta cheese mixture. Repeat layers. Top with final layer of noodles, sauce and remaining 1/2 cup of ricotta cheese.
Cover and bake at 350F for 40 minutes. Makes 8 servings.
Makes 8 servings

VEGETARIAN CHILI
Ten tbsp. Instant Protein Soy Mix
Four tbsp. olive oil

One cup onion, chopped
One can (14 1/2 oz.) Mexican style diced tomatoes
Two cans (14 1/2 oz.) vegetable broth
1/2 cup bulgar (cracked wheat)
1/2 cup green pepper chopped
One can (15 1/2 oz.) kidney beans
One cup frozen corn

1 1/2 tsp. chili powder
Salt to taste
Heat oil in a saucepan or Dutch oven and cook onions about 5 minutes or until soft. Stir in tomatoes, one can of vegetable broth, bulgur, and bell pepper; bring to a boil. Reduce heat and simmer covered stirring as needed until bulgur is tender about ten minutes. Add beans, corn, and chili powder. Mix second can of vegetable broth with the Instant Protein Soy Mix and then stir mixture into chili. For thinner chili, add additional vegetable broth or water, as desired. Makes 8 servings

ENEGY MOJITO
One lime peeled and quartered
8-10 fresh mint leaves, washed
One stick of green tea powder, (plain or pomegranate)
12-16 oz. filtered water or carbonated water
1/8 tsp. stevia drops or one Tbsp. sugar
Optional: 1-3 tbsp. orange or lime electrolyte powder*
Seven ice cubes or as desired

Method
Combine all ingredients except water and ice in a small bowl and grind together with a pestle or a mini-tart shaper until all lime juice has been squeezed out. Move all ingredients to a tall glass, then add ice and pour water over it. Stir and enjoy!

WAKE UP DETOX LEMONADE
Two cups filtered water...Get Clean water pitcher removes lead (cleansing)
One tsp. Vivix (anti-aging, metabolic boosting Resveterol)
One stick Shaklee 180 Energizing Tea (detoxing, with metabolic boosting EGCG, (a powerful green tea catechin)

One tbsp. Performance Orange or Lemon-Lime (hydrating)
One lime freshly squeezed
Stevia to taste
Stir then add ice. Best if enjoyed first thing in the morning, 30-60 minutes before breakfast. Also, make sure to swish water around in your mouth or brush your teeth immediately after drinking/eating any citrus fruits, pineapples, lemon water, or detox lemonade to wash the acids that can erode tooth enamel over time when consumed on a daily basis.

REFRESHING SUMMER TEA

In the morning boil three cups of water
Add ten alfalfa, one Energizing tea stick and three tbsp. of lemon lime Performance.
Let it sit to cool down. Then put it in a very nice jar with ten ice cubes and enjoy!

GET WELL TEA
Add ten alfalfa, one Energizing tea stick and three tbsp. of lemon lime Performance.
Let it sit to cool down. Then put it in a very nice jar with ten ice cubes and enjoy!
Add honey to taste. Sip from spoon or cup, stirring constantly.
Drink all the granules in your cup. For best results, drink another cup in 1/2 hour. Continue with one cup every hour until you are feeling better.
The granules are the result of crushing the following Shaklee products in a blender or coffee grinder.
Six Alfalfa, two Zinc, four Defend and Resist Complex (Echinacea, Black Elderberry, Larch Tree).
Four Garlic Complex (you may wish to take these separately rather than include them in the tea.
Four Mental Acuity Plus (includes Gingko, Biloba, Hawthorne, Bilberry, and Gota Kola and Rosemary).
Two Flavomax-remove from capsule
Four Osteo Matrix (includes Calcium, Phosphorous and Vitamin D.

Six Gentle Sleep Complex (includes Valerian, Passion Flower and German Chamomile Flower, Prune and Fig Powder).
Four Herblax (includes Anise, Alfalfa, Fennel, Blue Malva Flowers, Culvers Root Powder, Buckthorne Bark, Rhubarb Root, Senna, and Licorice)
Four Nutriferon
Four Stomach Soothing Complex (Peppermint and Ginger).
Three Vitamin C500mg (or 6-8 Chewable Vita C
Three tbsp. Performance
This tea can be kept in a jar when ready.

BE WELL TEA
To an eight ounce cup of hot water add:
1-2 tbsp. Performance
Three tablets Defend and Resist
Stir to dissolve. Sip and enjoy. Repeat in a few hours.
How to use GET WELL TEA
If you have a bug:
1. Drink the tea ten days straight. You can drink this several times a day to recover faster.
2. Then stop for five days.
3. If the bug is not gone do another ten days.
If the bug is gone but you work in an office or home where you are constantly exposed to germs you can follow the rotation below for keeping the bug away. To reduce your risk of getting a bug drink the tea four days a week then stop.
The reason for the rotation rather than every day is that Defend and Resist contain Echinacea which is an immune stimulant.
Constant stimulation of the immune system is not wise...therefore the rotation. If stomach is upset then adding one or two Stomach Soothing Complex will help.

www.ingramcontent.com/pod-product-compliance
Lightning Source LLC
Chambersburg PA
CBHW041525280526
45792CB00004B/1380